MY AMAZING Pregnancy ♡

(With Pregnancy Diary)

MY AMAZING Pregnancy

(With Pregnancy Diary)

Authored By,

Dr. Aliya Umaru

WINGS PUBLICATION INTERNATIONAL
WE GIVE WINGS TO YOUR DREAM!

Disclaimer

WINGS PUBLICATION INTERNATIONAL
WE GIVE WINGS TO YOUR DREAM!

Registered Office- 907-Sneh Nagar, Sapna Sangeeta Road, Agrasen Square, Indore – 452001 (M.P.), India

Website: http://www.wingspublication.com

Email: mybook@wingspublication.com

First Published by WINGS PUBLICATION 2023

Title : My amazing pregnancy

ISBN : 978-93-93966-72-8

LIMITS OF LIABILITY/DISCLAIMER OF WARRANTY

Author's Disclaimer

Although the author and publisher have made every effort to ensure that the information in this book was correct at press time, the author and publisher do not assume and hereby disclaim any liability to any party for any loss, damage, or disruption caused by errors or omissions, whether such errors or omissions result from negligence, accident, or any other cause.

Neither the author nor the publisher assumes any responsibility or liability whatsoever on behalf of the consumer or reader of this material. Any perceived slight of any individual or organization is purely unintentional.

The resources in this book are provided for informational purposes only and should not be used to replace the specialized training and professional judgment of a health care professional.

Neither the author nor the publisher can be held responsible for the use of the information provided within this book. Please always consult a trained professional before making any decision regarding treatment of yourself or others.

Dedication

This book is dedicated to my parents, who always believed in me.

And to my darlings - husband and children - who put up with my ambitions and told me that I could achieve anything if I put my mind to it.

To my cherished readers

Thank you for your purchase! Half of all the proceeds of this book will be donated to improve healthcare for pregnant women and their babies in impoverished communities all around the world. By buying this book, you have helped a woman somewhere, to have access to a safe pregnancy and birth.

Thank you.

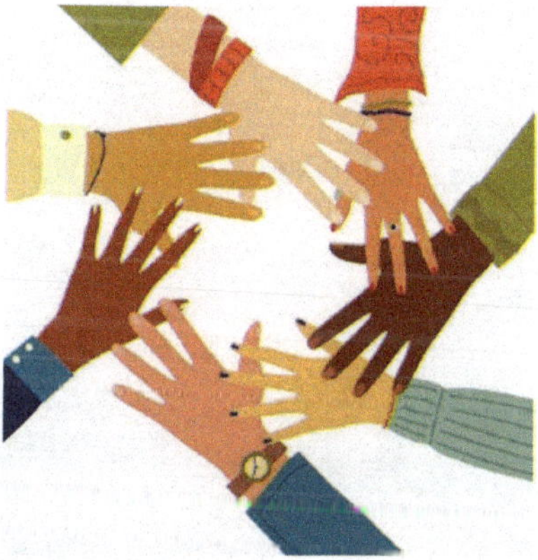

Introduction

Congratulations on taking the first step towards a safe, healthy, and enjoyable pregnancy, childbirth, and beyond!

Motivation for writing this book

We live in an era where people think they can find all the information they need at the touch of a button. While this is somewhat true, we also know this leads to information overload. Sometimes, information is overwhelming, unnecessary and can even be dangerous. Even when you come across reliable information, some of it is irrelevant. For instance, you can easily find pages of descriptions on how the embryo is growing, what milestones it reaches,how the organs and senses develop, etc. While this is all good for academic purposes, it is unlikely that knowing all this will help you achieve a healthy pregnancy and safe childbirth. We have chosen to add in information only if it translates to clinical decision-making. For example, we will only briefly discuss embryological organ formation when explaining the importance of taking folic acid.

Another dangerous phenomenon is information sharing. Naturally, women discuss their pregnancy and birth experiences and that of their friends, family, and associates. Again, while this is good and forms a part of our social connection, we must remember that all pregnancies are different, even for the same mother. So it can be extremely dangerous when women try to give or receive clinical advice based on personal, friend's, or sister's experience.

All the information that you need is highlighted in this book.It is based on the most up-to-date clinical practice and evidence-based medicine of world-class institutions. It is worth noting that all clinical care is (or at least should be) based on clinical guidelines. All world-class hospitals have agreed on guidelines that help clinicians diagnose, investigate, andmanage patients under their care. We have chosen to use the clinical guidelines of the United Kingdom, where the author has trained,and worked. Also,it is worth knowing that most clinical guidelines, regardless of the country of origin, are similar and based on the same evidence and research (as clinical researchers share their findings via various platforms such as international conferences, scientific papers, and journals). Further more, we buttress that they are only guidelines and do not replace the clinical judgement of your clinician. We highly encourage you to find a clinician who practices evidence based medicine and is also a good communicator, inorder to engage you in the decision about your care in pregnancy. It is your body and baby, after all!

There are also blank pages at the end of each chapter to write down your notes, thoughts, or questions for your healthcare provider, etc.

Our passion, mission, and vision is to empower women from all walks of life to take control and have enough knowledge, educating them on making informed decisions about the care they receive during their pregnancy and childbirth. Welcome to your new chapter! We promise to guide and support you.We would now like you to promise that you will engage with the process and begin your journey towards an amazing pregnancy and child birth.

Yours all the way,

Dr Aliya.

BLOOM

My Amazing Pregnany

How to use this book

This book has been structured in an easy-to-use format. A low-risk pregnancy (i.e., non-complicated pregnancy) on average lasts 40 weeks. Pregnancy is also divided into trimesters —the first, second, and third trimester being up till 13, 28, and 42 weeks, respectively.

The chapters in this book roughly represent eight weekly increments in an advancing pregnancy. Each chapter will describe a key change happening in your body and the clinical care you should receive at each point. It will also have a checklist to help you keep track of your progress.

You will find that some chapters are much longer than others because, in some weeks, more care is required than others in different stages or weeks of pregnancy.

Motivation first!

We would like you to stop for a moment before we begin and ask yourself, 'why?' Evidence suggests that whenever we know the 'why' for doing something, the how becomes easy. As a result, you are more likely to implement the amazing wealth of information that you now hold in your hands. So, to get the most out of this book, take a moment to complete the following exercise. For our future mamas who may have already been through pregnancy: use this chance to reflect on the nice things about your previous pregnancy (or pregnancies) and what you thought could have been different. For newbie mamas, this is the chance to write out your script and start your pregnancy journey on a good foot!

It is worth writing down your thoughts in the blank pages of your journal —it is for you to keep. Reflect on and revisit whenever you need a reminder. So, whip out your pen, and let's get writing!

Imagine your perfect pregnancy...

How will you find out? How will you feel (scared, anxious, excited, grateful, hopeful, etc.)?

How will you find your care providers?

What kind of relationship will you have with your obstetrician?

How will you feel as you bloom, feeling the life kicking inside of you?

How will you juggle work/family/home/relationships?

How will you feel when the pregnancy is coming to an end (whoop!) and the time to labour is near?

What were your preconceived ideas about pregnancy and labour before you read this book?

What do you look forward to most about pregnancy and labour, and what frightens you the most?

How will you put the knowledge you have now gained- to have your best possible pregnancy and childbirth?

TABLE OF CONTENTS

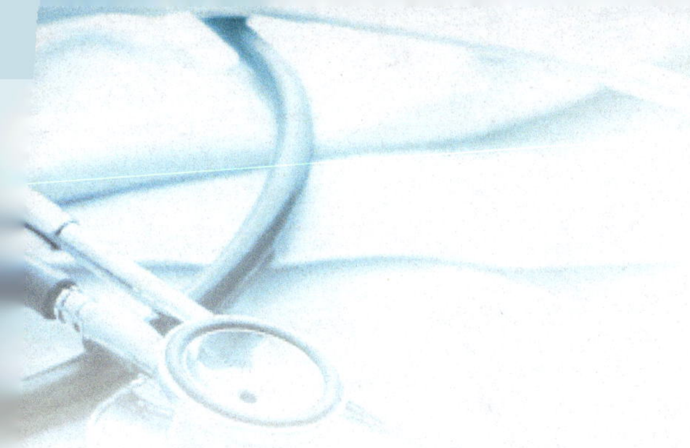

CHAPTER

One

Preconception

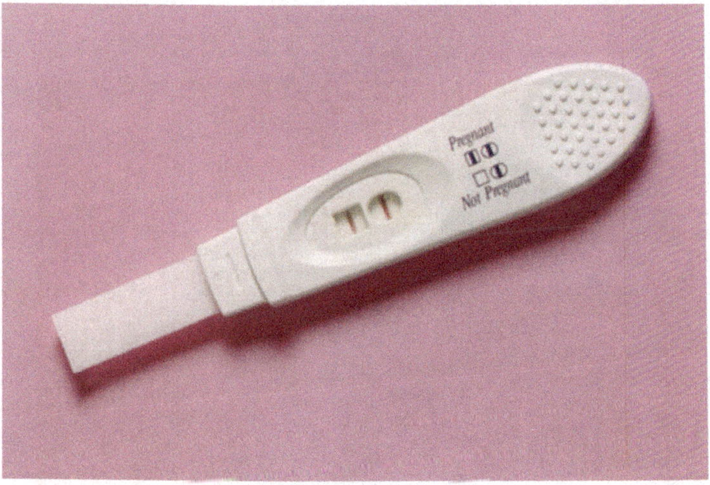

Hooray! Congratulations on deciding to become a mother. You might be at the stage in your life when you are ready —perhaps married and settled and ready for the next stages in life —to carry one within you, continuing your progeny. For those that are trying, we will discuss some important issues. For pregnant women, we will discuss how to navigate the first few weeks of pregnancy.

Optimise your health

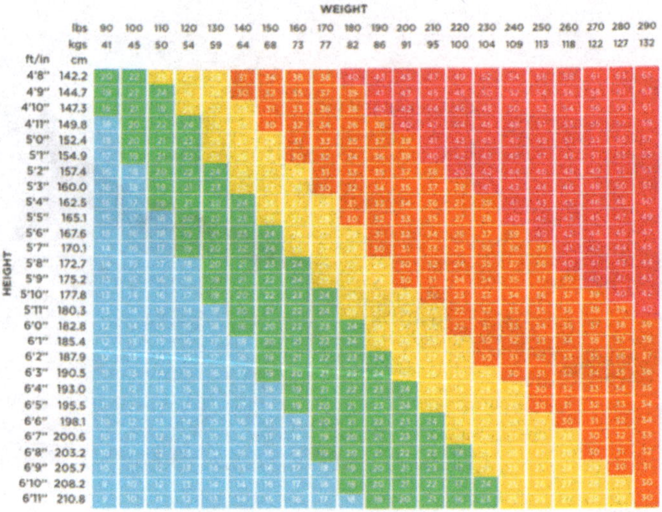

For an adult 20 years old or older, the **BMI ranges are the following:**

- **Underweight**: BMI is less than 18.5
- **Healthy weight**: BMI is between 18.5 and 24.9
- **Overweight**: BMI is between 25 and 29.9
- **Obesity**: BMI is 30 or more

Locate where your height and weight intersect to read your index on the BMI chart.

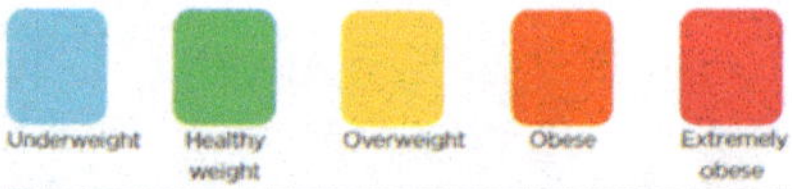

1. Being overweight

In the preconception stage of pregnancy, optimising your health before trying for a baby is the most important thing. If you are overweight (i.e., Body Mass Index of 30 and above), you should try to lose some weight. Even if coming down to a BMI of 30 is not achievable, shedding enough weight can go a long way towards reducing your risk of diabetes, Venous Thrombus Embolism (blood clots in your legs that can go to your lungs and be fatal), and congenital abnormalities in your baby. It will also improve your chances of achieving a natural birth. Most women add on an average of 15kg in pregnancy; hence, overweight women will be morbidly obese by the end of it. This has disastrous consequences for the pregnancy and general health later in life.

Being overweight also affects your fertility because being overweight means that you are more likely to have a condition called polycystic ovarian syndrome, where the ovaries have many small cysts.Women might also report abnormal periods and skin and hair changes, e.g., acne and the presence of facial hair.

2. Being underweight

Being underweight (BMI less than 18) is associated with reduced fertility. This is because underweight women have a reduced chance of ovulating, especially if this is associated with an eating disorder or excessive exercise. This would be presented as the absence of periods or having irregular periods. If you manage to fall pregnant and are underweight, this increases the risk of having a baby that does not grow well in pregnancy and may not reach its growth potential. This is known as Intrauterine Growth Restriction (IUGR) and has consequences for the baby's future physical and mental development.

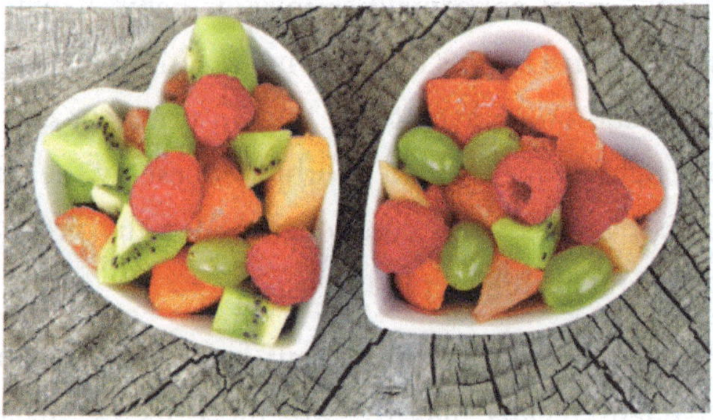

3. Chronic illnesses

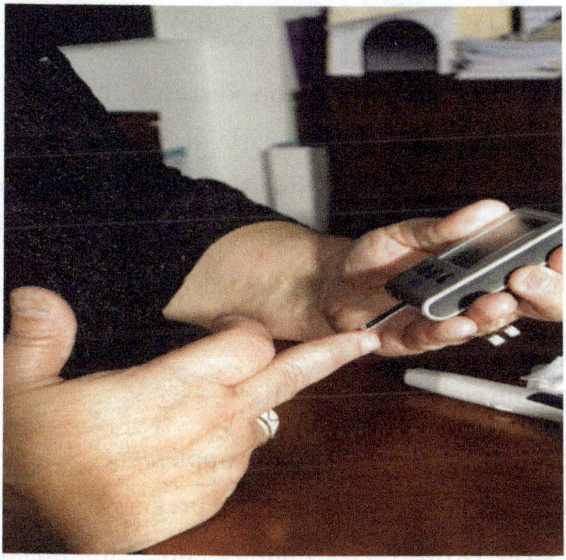

Suppose you suffer from any chronic disease (i.e., a disease that has lasted more than three months). In that case, it is highly recommended to make sure that things are under control and that you discuss your plans to become pregnant with your doctor or inform them that you are pregnant as soon as you find out. This is because most chronic illnesses will worsen by being pregnant and affect how your pregnancy progresses. The medication you use might also need adjusting or even changing. Many medications that will harm the foetus are associated with foetal abnormalities. However, you MUST not stop any medication without checking with your doctor or obstetrician first because you risk worsening your condition.The general principle is that the motheralways comes first!

Some of the most common diseases that can affect pregnancy are diabetes, heart disease, hypertension, kidney disease, sickle cell disease, anaemia, inflammatory bowel conditions, epilepsy, and mental health conditions such as depression, bipolar disorder, and schizophrenia. This is not an exhaustive list.

Taking the right supplements

There are many vitamins and supplements available for pregnant mothers. You can have a pregnancy supplement if you wish. However, the main essential vitamins that are necessary for a pregnant woman to take: Folic acid and vitamin D. Other important ones are:

- Vitamin C – protects the cells and helps keep them healthy. It is also found in a wide variety of fruit and vegetables such as oranges, red and green peppers, strawberries, broccoli, and many others.
- Calcium- It is vital for making your baby's bones and teeth. Sources include milk, cheese and yoghurt, tofu, green leafy vegetables such as rocket and watercress
- Iron – lack of iron leads to anaemia and fatigue. Good sources include lean meat, green leafy vegetables,

dried fruit, and nuts. Many breakfast cereals also contain added iron. Iron supplements are commonly prescribed to pregnant women.

1. Folic Acid?

Folic acid (or folate) is a B vitamin (B9) found mostly in dark green vegetables like broccoli and spinach, legumes such as beans and peas, and enriched grains.

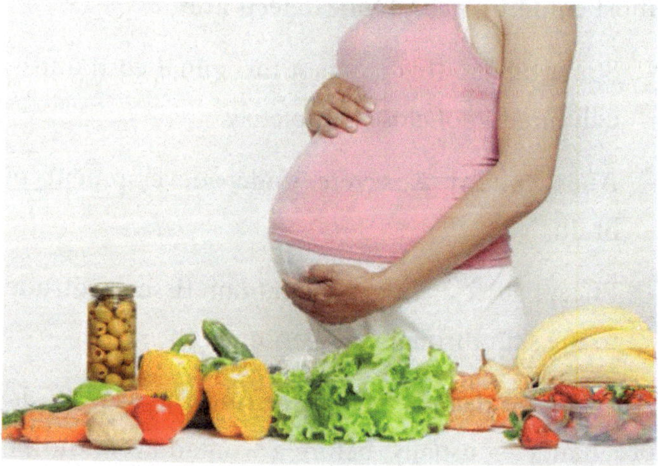

- **What Are the Benefits of Folic Acid?**

Pregnant women or women trying to become pregnant should get at least 400 micrograms (0.4 milligrams) of folic acid daily before conception and for at least three months afterwards. You can stop it when you get to 12 weeks because the brain and spinal cord would have developed. Studies show that this greatly reduces a baby's risk of serious neural tube defects. Some women who take medication for epilepsy or have had a previous baby with a Neural Tube Defect will need a higher dose of 5mg.

- **What Are Neural Tube Defects?**

Neural tube defects are congenital disabilities involving incomplete development of the brain and spinal cord. The most common neural tube defects are:

- Spina bifida: This is when the spinal cord and spinal column do not close completely.
- Anencephaly: A severe under development of the brain.
- Encephalocele: This is when brain tissue protrudes out to the skin through an opening in the skull.

All of these defects happen during the first 28 days of pregnancy — usually, before a woman even knows she's pregnant.

2. Vitamin D?

Vitamin D is known to play an important role in bone metabolism byregulating calcium and phosphate equilibrium. Vitamin D is produced by the body during exposure to sunlight but is also found in oily fish, eggs, and fortified food products.

Vitamin D deficiency is thought to be common among pregnant women in some populations. It can be associated with an increased risk of pre-eclampsia, gestational diabetes mellitus, preterm birth, and other conditions. Vitamin D supplementation during pregnancy improves maternal vitamin D status and may reduce the risk of pre-eclampsia, low birth weight, and preterm birth.

All pregnant women should take a 10 micrograms (or 400 IU) supplement of vitamin D each day.

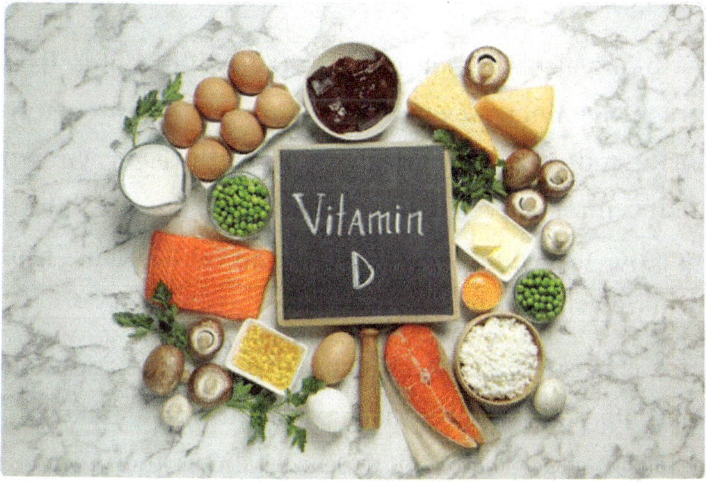

Lifestyle factors and herbal drugs

1. Smoking and drinking and recreational drugs

Women who smoke, drink alcohol or use recreational drugs are highly advised to quit as soon as possible with the help of qualified health care providers if necessary or if there is a problem with dependence.

Smoking during pregnancy increases the risk of health problems for developing babies, including preterm birth, low birth weight, and congenital abnormalities of the mouth and lip. Smoking during and after pregnancy also increases the risk of sudden infant death syndrome (SIDS).

Drinking alcohol, especially in the first three months of pregnancy, increases the risk of miscarriage, premature birth, and your baby having a low birthweight. Growth and central nervous system problems (e.g., low birth weight, behavioural problems) can also occur from drinking alcohol anytime during pregnancy.

This is because many substances pass easily through the placenta, so substances that a pregnant woman takes also reach the foetus. Recent research shows that smoking tobacco or marijuana, taking prescription pain relievers, or using illegal drugs during pregnancy is associated with double or even triple the risk of stillbirth. Regular use of some drugs can cause neonatal abstinence syndrome (NAS), in which the baby goes through withdrawal upon birth.

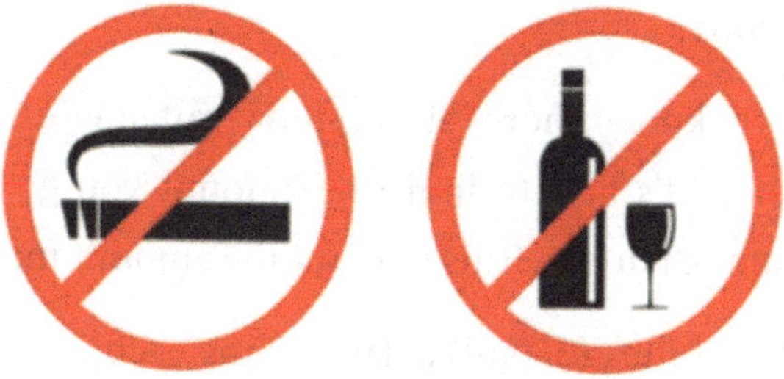

2. Caffeine

Caffeine slightly increases your blood pressure and heart rate and the amount of urine your body makes. Caffeine may cause you to feel jittery, have indigestion or have trouble sleeping. You may be especially sensitive to caffeine during pregnancy because it may take you longer to clear it from your body than if you weren't pregnant. It may also make you feel nauseous or lightheaded.

When you have caffeine during pregnancy, it passes through the placenta to your baby. The placenta grows in your uterus (womb), supplying the baby with food and oxygen through the umbilical cord.

You may have heard that too much caffeine can cause miscarriage (when a baby dies in the womb before 20 weeks of pregnancy), preterm birth (birth that happens before 37 weeks of pregnancy is completed), or low birth weight (when your baby is born weighing less than five pounds, eight ounces). Some studies say this is true, and others don't.

Until we know more about how caffeine can affect pregnancy, it's best to limit the amount you get to 200 milligrams each day. This is about the amount in:

Two mugs of tea (350ml) a day – 75mg each.

Two mugs of instant coffee – 100mg each.

Five cans of cola – 40mg each.

Two energy drinks (250ml) - 80mg each.

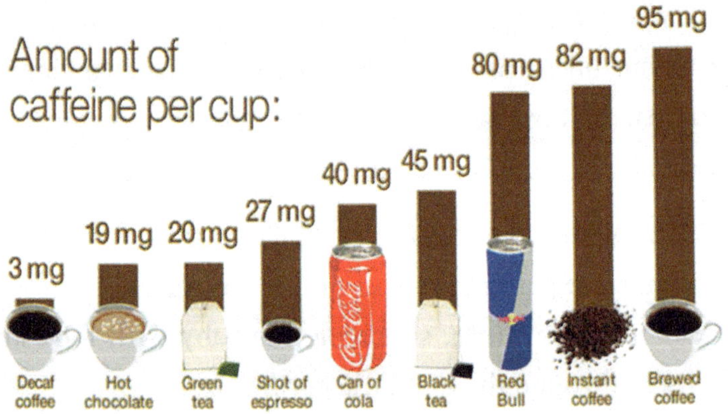

3. Herbal medications

Do you take any other medications, e.g., herbal supplements? This could be in the form of powders, teas, tablets, etc. Most have not been well-studied regarding their safety and ability to work as they are advertised. Also, there are no standards for ingredients and strength. Be mindful of product claims such as "works better than [a prescription drug]," "totally safe," or has "no side effects." Be aware that the term "natural" does not mean safe.

Levels of active ingredients in herbal preparations depend on the growth and harvest conditions, plant parts used (e.g., root, stem, flower, or bark), and how they are made into supplements.

Some herbal products might contain contaminants such as metals (lead, arsenic, and mercury), pesticides, other chemicals, or microorganisms (e.g., fungi or bacteria). They may even contain other products not listed on the label.

Does taking herbal products increase the chance of congenital disabilities?

Every pregnancy starts with a 3-5% chance of having a congenital disability. This is called the background risk. There is limited information on the use of most herbal products during pregnancy. Information on products that contain multiple herb ingredients is very hard to study for safety. There are concerns about interactions between ingredients in these products and other medications an individual may be taking and concerns over harmful substances not noted on the label.

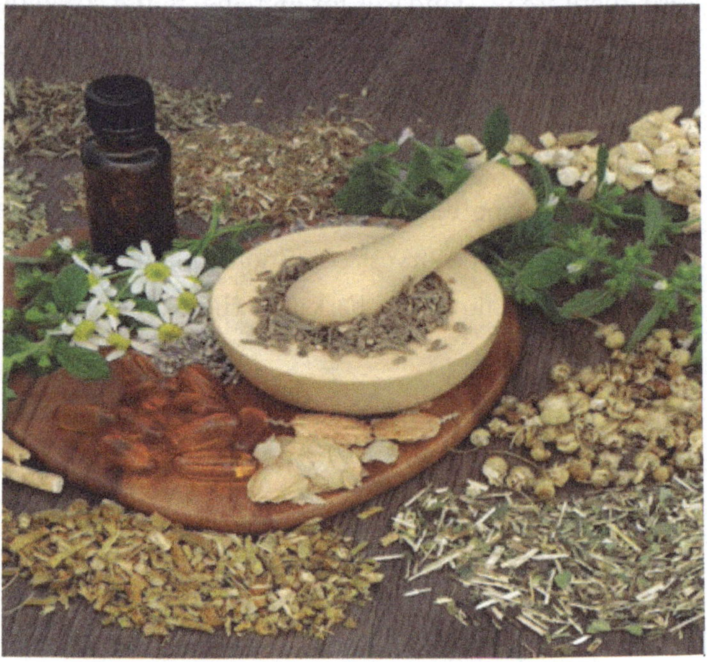

Does taking herbal products during pregnancy increase the chance of other pregnancy-related problems?

Some products have been shown to bring on labour, cause pregnancy loss, hormone imbalance, or uterine contractions. Read the label on the product and discuss each ingredient with your healthcare provider.

Does taking herbal products during pregnancy affect future behaviour or learning for the child?

Many herbal products have not been studied on possible long-term effects on the developing baby. Therefore, it is not known if there is or is not any increased chance of long-term problems in behaviour or learning for the baby.

Vaccinations in pregnancy

Some vaccines, such as the inactivated seasonal flu vaccine and the whooping cough vaccine, are recommended during pregnancy to protect the health of you and your baby. An inactivated vaccine does not contain a live version of the virus it protects against.

Vaccines not usually advised in pregnancy (live vaccines)

If a vaccine uses a live version of the virus, such as the MMR vaccine, you'll usually be advised to wait until after your baby is born before you get vaccinated. This is because there's a potential risk that live vaccines could cause your unborn baby to become infected. However,there's no evidence that any live vaccine causes congenital disabilities.

Live vaccines include:

- BCG (vaccination against tuberculosis)
- MMR (measles, mumps, and rubella)

- Oral polio (which forms part of the 5-in-1 vaccine given to infants)
- Oral typhoid
- Yellow fever

Recommended Vaccinations in pregnancy:

1. Rubella

   It is important for every woman considering getting pregnant to be immune to rubella (MMR vaccine). If you are not pregnant yet, you can get this vaccine, but you should wait for a month before conceiving. If you are already pregnant, you will have to wait until your baby is born.

what can happen if a pregnant woman gets rubella?

Congenital rubella syndrome (CRS) is a condition that occurs in a developing baby in the womb whose mother is infected with the rubella virus. Pregnant women who contract rubella are at risk of miscarriage or stillbirth. Their developing babies are at risk for severe congenital disabilities with devastating, lifelong consequences. CRS can affect almost everything in the developing baby's body.

The most common congenital disabilities from CRS can include:

- Deafness
- Cataracts
- Heart defects
- Intellectual disabilities
- Liver and spleen damage
- Low birth weight
- Skin rash at birth

2. Coronavirus (COVID-19) vaccine.

   If you're pregnant or think you might be, you can have the coronavirus (COVID-19) vaccine.

Preferably, you should have the Pfizer/BioNTech or Moderna vaccine. This is because they've been more widely used during pregnancy in other countries and have not caused any safety issues.

You can be vaccinated against coronavirus (COVID-19) if:

- You're pregnant or think you might be.
- You're breastfeeding.
- You're trying for a baby or might get pregnant in the future.

There's no evidence that the COVID-19 vaccines have any effect on your chances of becoming pregnant, and there's no need to avoid getting pregnant after being vaccinated.

Which vaccine is better in pregnancy?

If you're pregnant and have not had a COVID-19 vaccine yet, you should have the Pfizer/BioNTech or Moderna vaccine.

These vaccines have been more widely used during pregnancy in other countries, and no safety concerns have been identified.

If you've already had the Oxford/AstraZeneca vaccine for your first dose and did not have any serious side effects, you should have it again for your second dose.

The vaccines cannot give you or your baby COVID-19.

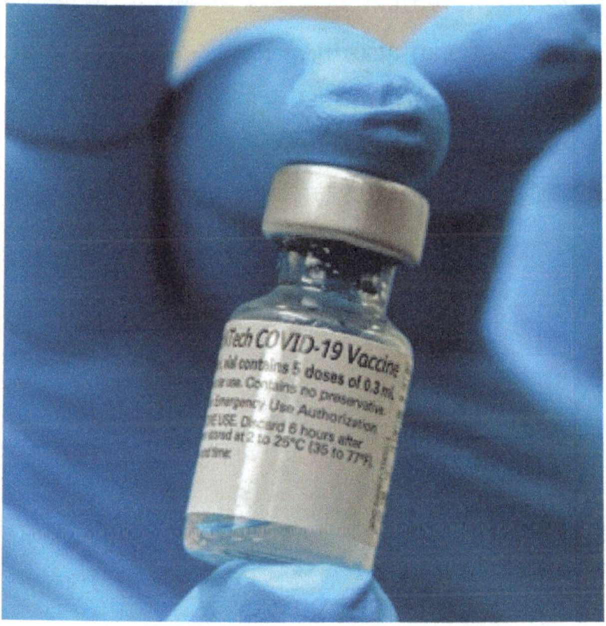

Effects of COVID-19 in pregnancy

Although it's very rare for pregnant women to become seriously ill if they get COVID-19, it may be more likely later in pregnancy. If this happens, there's a small chance your baby may be born early, or you may be advised to give birth earlier than your due date.

While the chances of having a stillbirth are low, there is some emerging evidence that the risk may be higher if you have COVID-19 at the time of birth.

It's important to follow advice to stop the spread of COVID-19 throughout your pregnancy. Especially when you're more than 28 weeks pregnant (in your third trimester), you can also have the COVID-19 vaccine to help protect you and your baby.

Checklist- preconception and early pregnancy

My BMI is 18-30 (Or I am taking an active step to make it so).

I have been given the go-ahead by my doctor to try for pregnancy (and my medications have been reviewed).

I have started taking a 10-mcg vitamin D supplement.

I have started taking a 400-mcg folic acid supplement.

I have stopped smoking, alcohol, and recreational drugs (or seeking the right help if applicable).

I have stopped taking all herbal remedies and supplements.

I have limited my caffeine intake to 200mg a day.

My vaccinations are up-to-date, and I am immune to rubella.

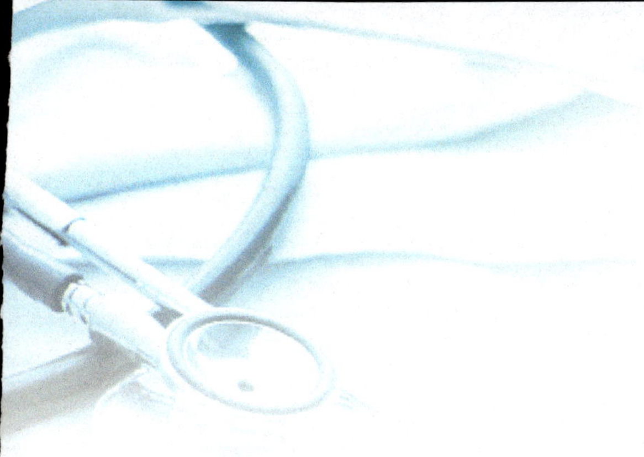

CHAPTER

Two

Week 4-12

Your baby is the size of these fruits!

At each appointment, you should have a BP check, and urine should be checked for signs of infection (leukocytes and nitrites), diabetes (glucose), and pre-eclampsia (protein).

At this stage, you should be looking to have your first antenatal (booking) appointment with a midwife or an obstetrician by 10+0 weeks of pregnancy. At this visit, the appointments for the duration of your pregnancy should be determined. You should also be categorised as a low-risk or high-risk pregnancy. This manual will mostly cover low-risk pregnancies as extra coverage will be required for high-risk conditions. However, we will introduce some of the most common conditions in pregnancy, such as pre-eclampsia.

How many appointments should I need?

A woman in her first pregnancy (nulliparous) is recommended to have10 appointments. A woman in her subsequent pregnancies (multiparous) is recommended to have 7 appointments.

What should I expect in my first antenatal visit?

1. The full history of your previous pregnancies, medical conditions, and family history will determine what care you receive in your current pregnancy.
2. Blood tests: This is to check for:

- HIV
- Syphilis
- Hepatitis B
- Sickle cell
- Thalassaemia
- Full-Blood Count and Blood group and Rhesus status (i.e., Rhesus positive or negative)

3. Measure your height, weight, body mass index, and Blood Pressure.

4. Risk assessment for specific conditions: Your doctor should also assess your risk of the following conditions because if you are at high risk, you should be offered further management/care.

- Gestational diabetes (you should be offered screening at 24+0 and 28+0 weeks). All women of Black ethnic origin fall into this category.
- Pre-eclampsia. (If you are considered at risk, you should be offered 150mg of Aspirin at night.) (You should take this from 12 weeks until 38 weeks of pregnancy.)
- Foetal growth restriction. (If you are at risk, you should be offered growth scans of your baby at 28, 32, 36, and 40 weeks respectively)
- Venous thromboembolism. (If you are at risk, you should be offered blood thinning injections from 28 weeks of pregnancy or earlier depending on your level of risk.)

Screening for foetal abnormality

In most countries, pregnant women are offered a screening test for Down's syndrome, Edwards' syndrome, and Patau's syndrome between 10 and 14 weeks of pregnancy. This is to assess your chances of having a baby with one of these conditions. It is done by calculating your baby's risk based on a combination of an ultrasound scan with a blood test and your age.It will give either a high or a low-risk result.

If your first screen has shown that your baby has a higher chance of having Down's syndrome, Edwards' syndrome, or Patau's syndrome, this doesn't mean your baby definitely has one of these chromosomal conditions.

Further testing can give you more accurate information about how likely it is that your baby may have any of these conditions. These include:

-A further screening test - non-invasive prenatal testing, known as NIPT.

-A diagnostic test - chorionic villus sampling (CVS) or amniocentesis.

It is important to remember that no screening test is 100% accurate.

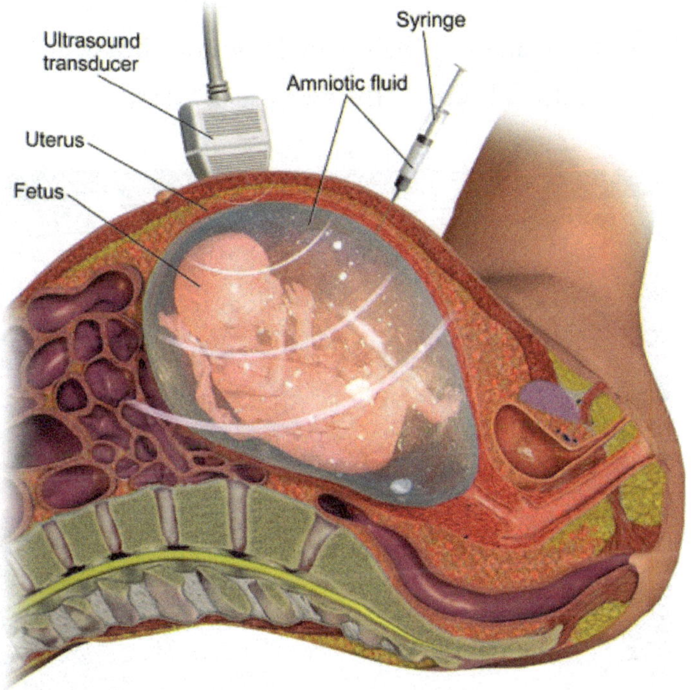

Amniocentesis image

The 'Dating' Ultrasound scan.

Your first scan of the baby should be done between 11+2 weeks and 14+1 weeks. The purpose of this scan is:

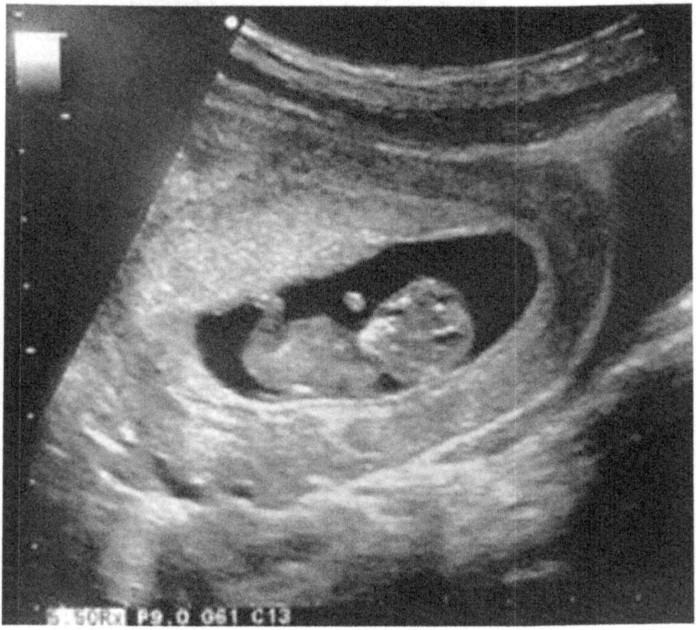

- Detect multiple pregnancies and determine gestational age (and therefore calculate your due date.This is necessary if you do not deliver by your expected due date).
- It can also be used by trained professionals to detect certain conditions, e.g., Down's syndrome.

Checklist:Week 4-12

I have had my blood tests.

My full medical, family, and previous obstetric history have been reviewed.

I have had my dating USS.

My appointments have been booked, and I know whom to contact in an emergency.

I know if I will have a low-risk or high-risk pregnancy care package.

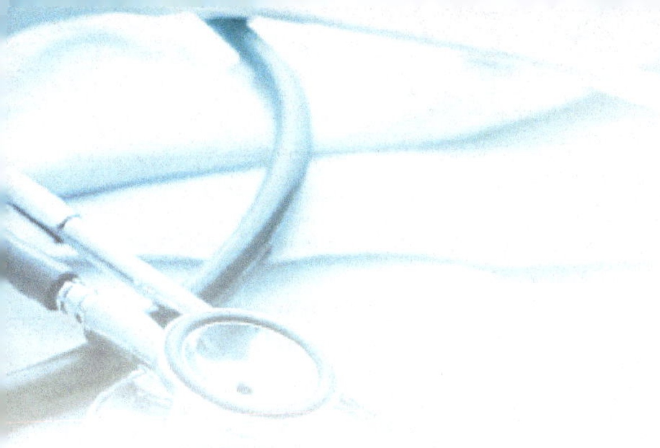

CHAPTER

Three

Week 12-20

20 WEEKS

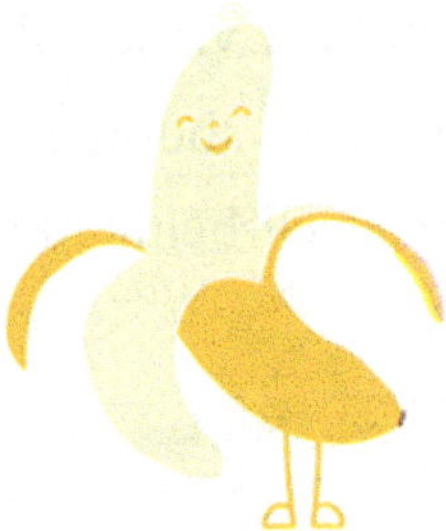

Your baby is as big as a...BANANA!

At each appointment, you should have a BP check, and urine should be checked for signs of infection (leukocytes and nitrites), diabetes (glucose), and pre-eclampsia (protein).

You should be offered an ultrasound scan to:

- Screen for foetal anomalies.
- Determine the placental location. (If the placenta is low, you should be offered another scan to check for placental location at 32 or 36 weeks.)
- Results of any tests from previous appointments.
- You get to hear your baby's heartbeat for the first time! From 16 weeks onwards, your midwife or doctors should listen to your baby's heartbeat with a sonicaid.

However, some places still use the traditional Pinard to listen to the foetal heart. If there are any concerns, then you will be offered a CTG (Cardiotocography). A CTG is a continuous recording of the fetal heart rate obtained via an ultrasound transducer placed on the mother's abdomen. It is used as a method of assessing fetal well-being in pregnancy.

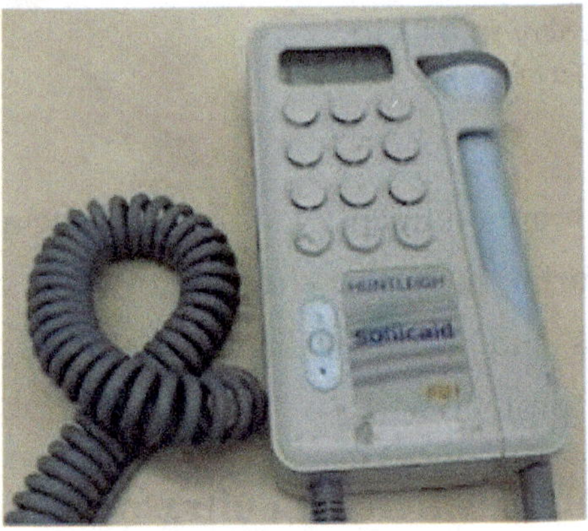

Sonicaid

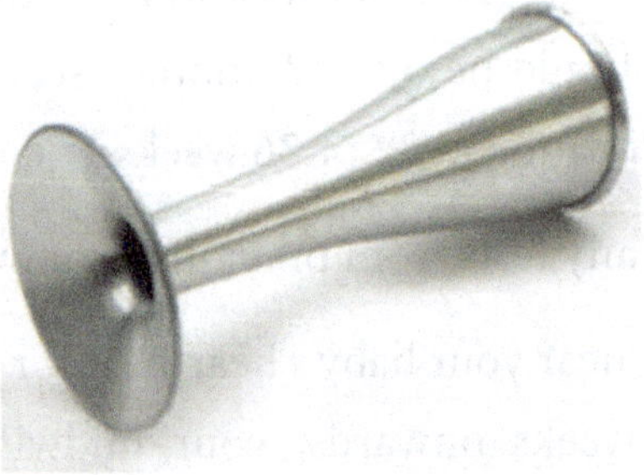

Pinard

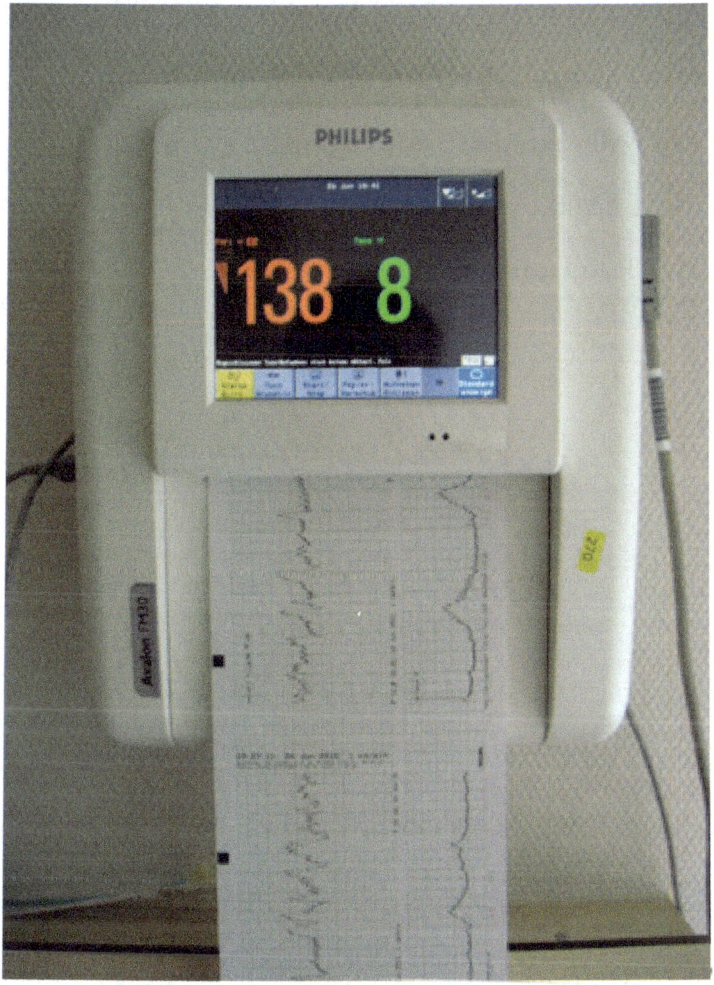

CTG machine

Checklist: Week 12-20

I have had a USS to check for foetal abnormalities.

I know the position of my placenta.

I have had the results of all my blood tests.

My BP and urine and normal.

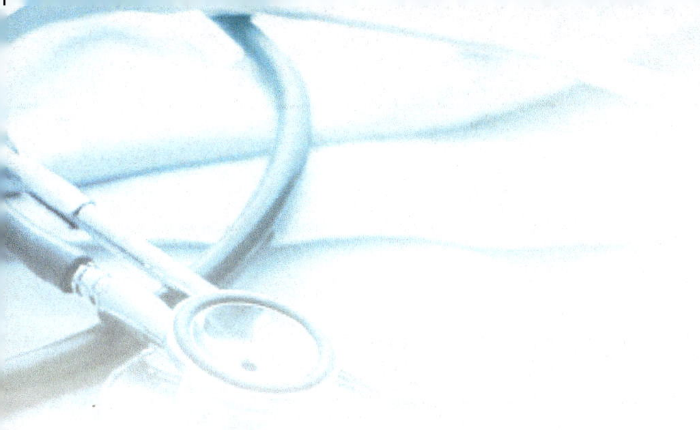

CHAPTER

Four

Week 20-28

At each appointment, you should have a BP check, and urine should be checked for signs of infection (leukocytes and nitrites), diabetes (glucose), and pre-eclampsia (protein).

At this stage, you should be offered:

1. A repeat blood test to check full-blood count, blood group, and antibodies.
2. To prevent the risk of Rhesus disease, Anti-D prophylaxis should be given to rhesus-negative women —this would consist of one or two injections of Anti D. Rhesus disease is a condition where antibodies in a pregnant woman's blood destroy her baby's blood cells. It's also known as haemolytic disease of the foetus and newborn (HDFN).

Rhesus disease doesn't harm the mother, but it can cause the baby to become anaemic and develop jaundice. This is likely to happen not in the first pregnancy but in subsequent ones.

3. An Oral Glucose tolerance test to screen for the presence of gestational diabetes between 24 and 28 weeks should be offered to all Black and Asian women.

4. Symphysis fundal height measurement (SFH) at each antenatal appointment after 24+0 weeks and auscultation (listening) of the foetal heart: if there are concerns about a small or large baby, you should then be referred for a growth scan.

Furthermore, you should contact maternity services if you have any concerns about her baby's movements (i.e., feel as if the baby was not moving as well as it normally does) after 24+0 weeks.

Checklist: Week 20-28

I have had repeat blood tests.

I have had my GTT.

My SFH has been measured and is normal.

I have heard my baby's heartbeat.

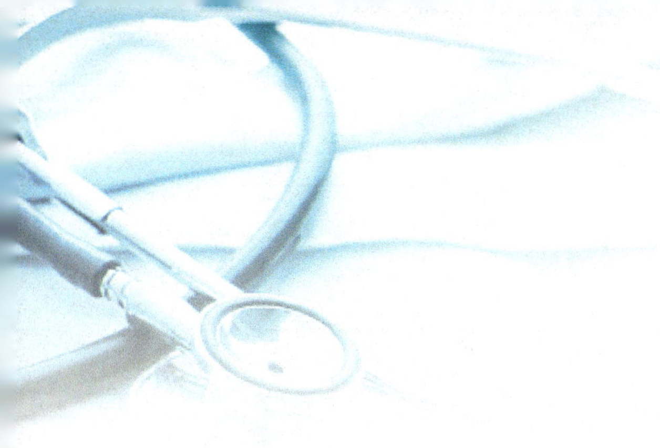

CHAPTER

Five

Week 28-36

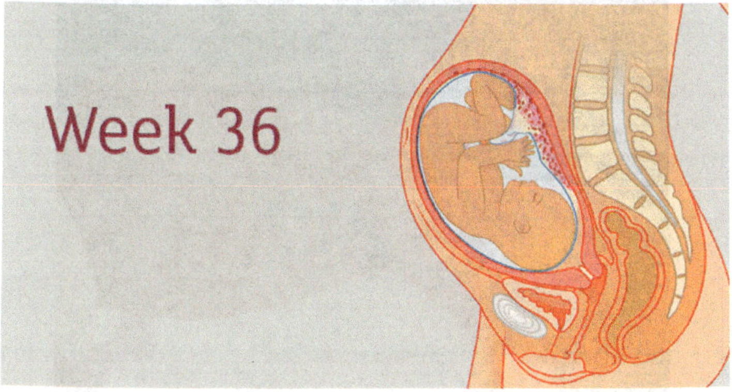

At each appointment, you should have a BP check, and urine should be checked for signs of infection (leukocytes and nitrites), diabetes (glucose), and pre-eclampsia (protein).

Also add that in some parts of the world, women might routinely be offered growth scans instead of SFH measurements.

1. Sleep position from 28 weeks

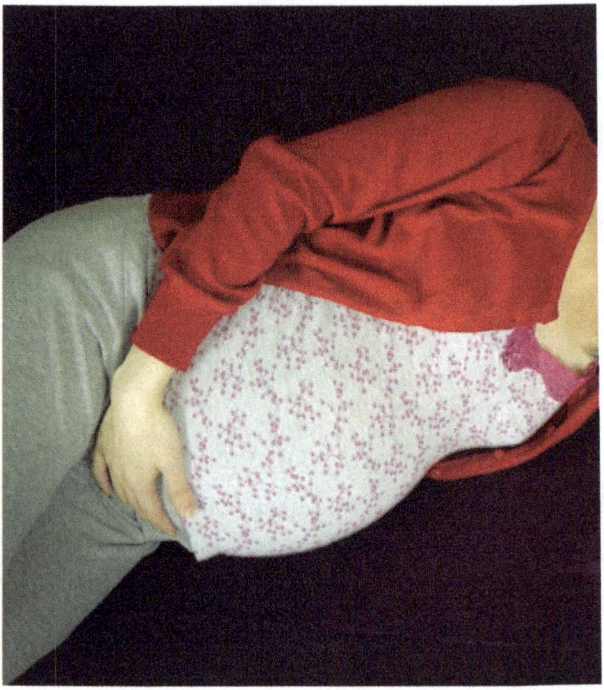

It is advised to avoid going to sleep on your back after 28 weeks of pregnancy. This is because there may be a link between going to sleep on your back and stillbirth in late pregnancy (after 28 weeks).

2. Breech or cephalic (head down)?

It is not uncommon for babies to be in the breech position (bottom down). 20% of babies are breech at 28 weeks, and most babies turn spontaneously, resulting in an incidence of 3 to 4% at term. So, we only start to think about what to do if your baby is breech at 36 weeks.

3. **At this stage, you should be offered:**

Abdominal palpation at all appointments after 36+0 weeks to identify possible breech presentation for women with a singleton pregnancy.

If a breech presentation is suspected on abdominal palpation, you should have an ultrasound scan to confirm the presentation.

For women with an uncomplicated singleton pregnancy with breech presentation confirmed after 36+0 weeks:

You should discuss the different options available and their benefits, risks, and implications, including:

- External cephalic version (ECV) (to turn the baby from bottom to head down)
- Breech vaginal birth
- Elective caesarean birth

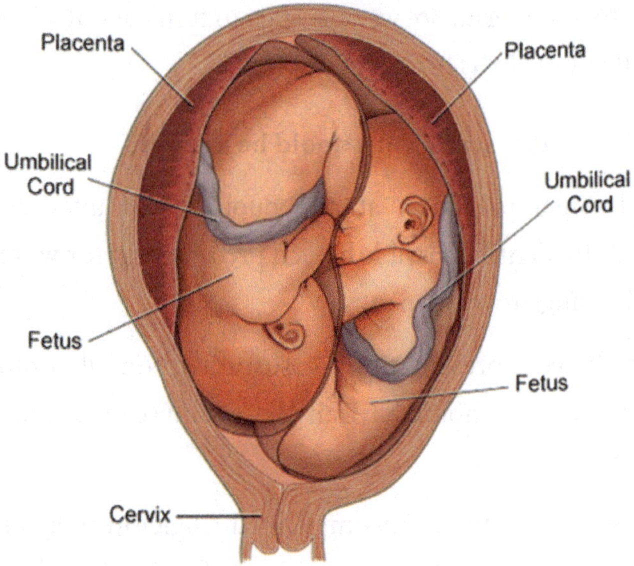

Twins- One breech, one cephalic.

Checklist: Week 28-36

I have checked my blood tests and have tablets for anaemia (if needed).

My baby is growing normally on scan/SFH measurements.

I know what to do/whom to call if my baby's movements are reduced.

I have had my GTT (test for diabetes), and action is taken if it is abnormal.

I know my baby's position at 36 weeks.

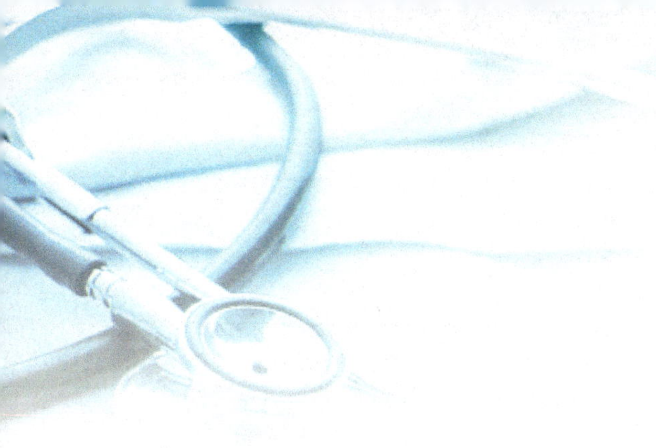

CHAPTER

Six

Week 36-42

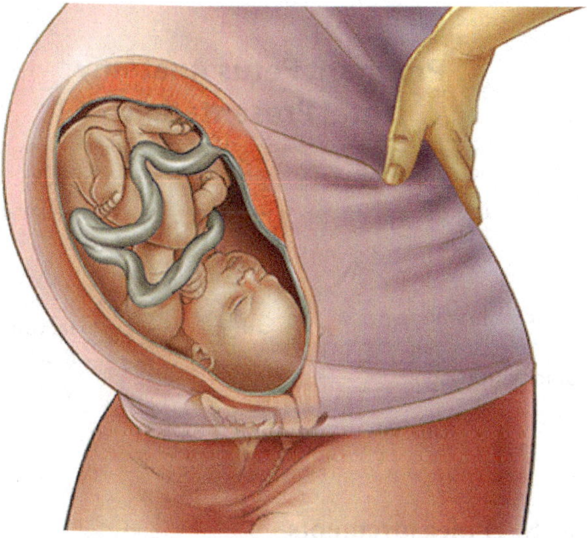

At each appointment, you should have a BP check, and urine should be checked for signs of infection (leukocytes and nitrites), diabetes (glucose), and pre-eclampsia (protein).

1. Placenta and foetal presentation

At this stage, if you had a low-lying placenta at your anomaly scan at around 20 weeks, you should have another scan to recheck the position of the placenta. The scan will confirm that the placenta is no longer low, and the baby is head down (or sometimes you can be allowed to deliver with a low placenta if the foetal head is below the leading edge of the placenta). If both have been checked, you are all set to await the onset of labour!

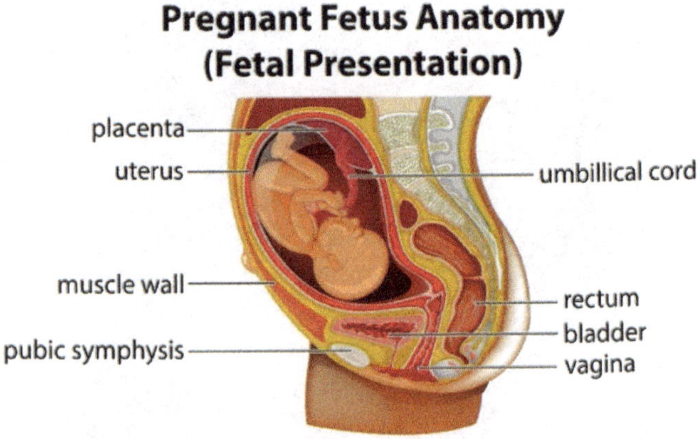

2. SFH measurements

You should also continue to have SFH measurements (starting from around 26 weeks) every two weeks, preferably by the same person, to reduce the risk of humans in error. You should also monitor your baby closely for a reduction in how they move and report this as soon as possible to your care provider.

3. Reduced foetal movements and CTG monitoring

If you have reduced foetal movements, you should be offered a CTG monitoring of the baby after 28 weeks. Cardiotocography (CTG) is a continuous recording of the foetal heart rate obtained via an ultrasound transducer placed on the mother's abdomen. CTG is widely used in pregnancy to assess foetal well-being, predominantly in pregnancies with increased risk of complications.

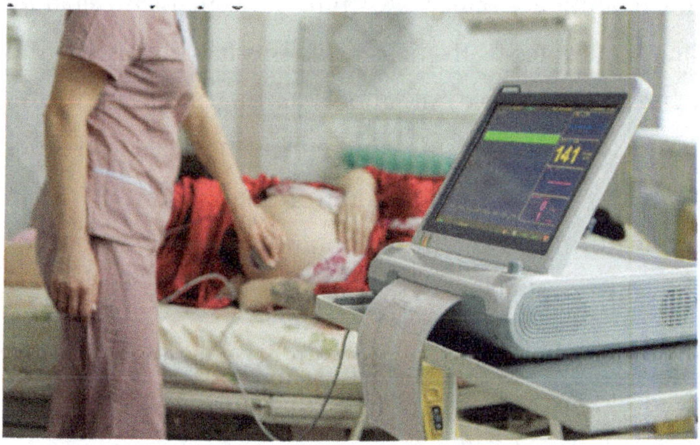

If you have a second episode of reduced foetal movements, you should be offered a growth scan if you have not had one in the last twoweeks. If you have reduced foetal movements after 38-39 weeks, you should be offered an induction of labour or a stretch and sweep of the cervix to stimulate labour.

4. Cervical or membrane sweeps

You can also consider having membrane sweeps from 39-40 weeks.

5. What is a membrane sweep?

Membrane sweeping involves your midwife or doctor placing a finger just inside your cervix (neck of the womb) and making a circular, sweeping movement to separate the membranes from the cervix. This has been shown to increase the chances of labour starting naturally within the next 48 hours and can reduce the need for other methods of induction of labour. It may be carried out at home, during an antenatal appointment, at your surgery, or in the hospital.

The procedure may cause slight discomfort, slight bleeding, or a 'show' and tightening of the womb. These are normal and will not cause any harm to you or your baby. It will not increase the chance of your baby getting an infection.

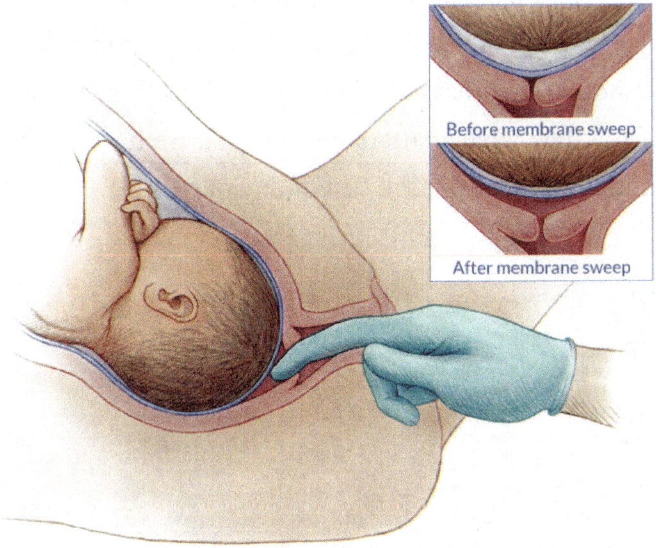

Membrane sweeping is not recommended if your waters have broken.

Well-done! You are nearly there! All nausea, pain, injections, appointments, anxiety are about to end, and you will be meeting your baby soon!

6. Preparing for labour

You might start having more anxiety about the labour. It is important to know what to expect, what is normal, and how labour should progress naturally. This will help you relax and have a better chance of achieving a successful birth. Nevertheless, also remember that no one canaccurately predict which babies will be successfully delivered through the vagina and who will need delivery by a Caesarean section, so do not be disappointed if you do not entirely have the birth you wished for. At the end of the day, what matters most is that we have a healthy mother and baby at the end of the journey.

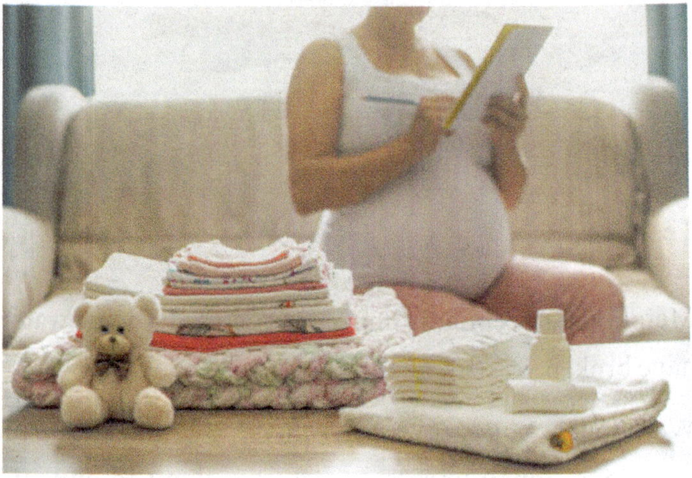

You should, at this stage, think about your birth plan and what some of your wishes will be and discuss them with your care provider to see how much of it can be accommodated. Some of the things you should ask now to avoid disappointment are:

- Your option for pain relief in labour.
- Birth partner and how many would be allowed.

- Options for who can be allowed in case you need a Caesarean section.
- What the hospital provides (e.g., meals).
- Discuss what you wish to bring to the hospital, e.g., your TENS machine, essential oils.
- How long you should expect to stay in hospital (if all goes well!).
- Discuss positions for delivery with your doctor/ midwife.

7. Beyond 40 weeks

So, it seems as if your baby likes it in there and does not want to come out!

At weeks 40 and 41 of antenatal visits, nulliparous women should undergo a vaginal examination for membrane sweeping.

At week 41 of antenatal visit, parous women should under go a vaginal examination for membrane sweeping.

However, there is some new evidence that pregnant mothers from black ethnic groups should be offered Induction of Labour (IOL) from 39 weeks (and so cervical sweeps from around 38 weeks).

We would encourage that you discuss this with your health care provider and see which one would suit you and your pregnancy more.

Discussions on labour and delivery will be covered in the sequel to this book — 'My amazing labour'. See you there!

Checklist: Week 36-42

My baby is head down, and the placenta is not low (or I have discussed this with my doctor).

I have discussed my birth preferences and know what to expect in labour.

I have discussed what the options are if I go over my due date.

I know what to do/whom to call if my baby's movements are reduced.

I have packed my bags, and I am ready to go! (P.S- you can use one of the blank pages to write out a list of what you might require to pack in your hospital bag).

Can You Help?

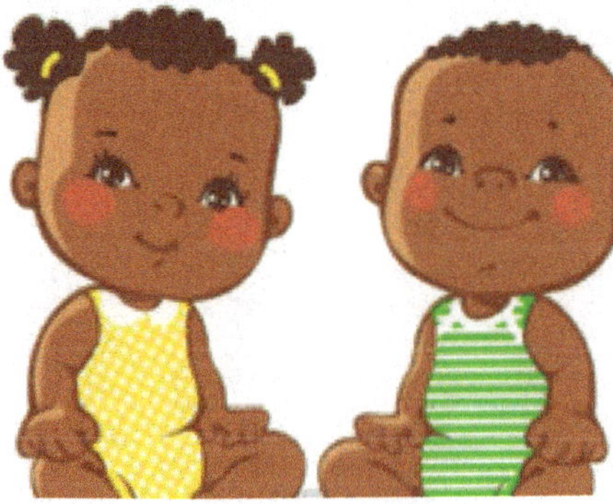

Thank You for Reading My Book!

I really appreciate all of your feedback, and I love hearing what you have to say.

I need your input to make the next version of this book and my future books better.

Please leave me an honest review on Amazon letting me know what you thought of the book.

Thanks so much!

Dr. Aliya.

***

Made in the USA
Monee, IL
03 November 2026

67386686R00066